Jailhouse Strong

Jailhouse Strong

■ ■ ■

Tactical Shield Training

Josh Bryant and Adam benShea

Jailhouse Strong: Tactical Shield Training JoshStrength, LLC and Adam benShea

Copyright © 2019

All rights reserved, including file sharing and the right to reproduce this work, in whole or any part, in any form. All inquiries must be directed to Josh Bryant and Adam benShea and have approval from both authors.

Table of Contents

Introduction	1
The Importance of Neck Training	5
Neck Function	9
Neck Rotations	12
Neck Flexions	14
Neck Extensions	16
Neck Lateral Flexions	17
Final Thoughts	19
The Total Trap Development Program	20
About the Movement: Farmer's Walk	23
About the Movement: Hise Shrugs	26
About the Movement: Face Pulls	27
About the Movement: Incline Dumbbell Shrugs	29
About the Movement: Band Y-Raises	30
About the Movement: Straight Arm Dip Shrugs	31
About the Movement: T3 Raises	32
About the Movement: One-Arm Barbell Shrugs	34
About the Movement: Suspended Isometric Kettlebell Shrugs	35
About the Movement: Gittleson Shrugs	37
About the Movement: Half-Mile Carry	38

The Jailhouse Strong Tactical Shield Training
(TST) Program 39
   Extra Meat for Extra Training 58
      Zen and the Lost Art of Isometrics 59
      Isometrics for the Front Neck Muscles 59
      Isometrics for the Back Neck Muscles 59
      Isometrics for the Side Neck Muscles
      (Neck Lateral Flexors) 59
   Neck Training for Combat Sports 60
   Nod If You Want a Stronger Neck 60
   Walk Tall 61
   Conclusion 62

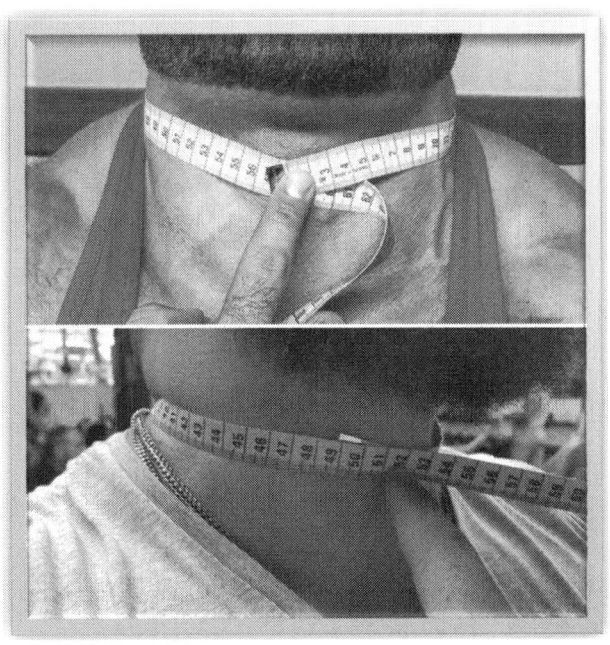

Figure 1. Baptiste Deodati added nearly 3 inches to an already 19 inch neck with TST.

Introduction

In the ancient Mediterranean world, there was a prominent city-state known as Lacedaemon which rose to military prominence because of their fiercely trained warriors. We know them as the Spartans.

Upon completion of the *agoge*—the rigorous education and training required for every male Spartan citizen—the young Spartan was eligible to become an active member of the Lacedaemonian army.

Conflict inside of Sparta (as Lacedaemon became known based on the name of its main settlement) and between other Greek city-states was frequent. The historian Thucydides tells us that before a Spartan man went off to war, his wife would hand him his shield (*hoplon*) and say: "With this, or upon this." In other words, a warrior could only return to Sparta with his shield in hand or dead upon it.

The idea was that in the midst of battle, should fear overtake a Spartan and he run from the fighting, the first thing he would drop would be his shield. Coming home without his shield would be a telltale sign that cowardice had broken the Spartan warrior. This was unacceptable. At Jailhouse Strong, we recognize the struggle with fear, but we cannot abide by the willingness to be bent, bowed, and broken by cowardice.

So, never leave your shield.

A developed and muscled neck serves to protect your body, back, and brain from trauma, damage, and injury.

Your neck is your shield. Build it, develop it, and don't leave home without it. If ancient tales from antiquity don't resonate with you, remember: Bulging biceps might save you from dateless Saturday nights, but a strong neck can save your ass.

Neck training is a necessity, not a luxury, for football, boxing, MMA, rugby, the unexpected bar fight, and any combat sport where blows to the head are common. A strong neck can reduce the likelihood of a concussion because it diminishes brain rattling after a big hit.

When it comes to developing your neck as a shield of protection, the modern-day tactical athlete is no exception. Whether you're a warfighter deployed in Afghanistan, a corrections officer in China's Chongzhou prison, or a beat cop working the streets of Gary, Indiana, a strong neck can help to keep you safe.

Beyond injury prevention, a strong, muscular neck is a fundamental piece in a symmetrical physique that can help remedy postural abnormalities. It can also aid strength gains throughout the entire upper body. As world-renowned strength coach Charles Poliquin explained it: "The stronger the neck, the faster the strength gains in the upper extremities."

On a practical level for those in the service or considering serving, the U.S. Army, Navy, and Marine Corps use a basic height-weight body mass index tool as an initial assessment. Those who exceed weight limits get "taped." This means that men are measured at the neck and waist and women are measured at the neck, waist, and hips. For both, the neck measurement is subtracted from the other measurements in an equation designed to determine "circumference value." Those results are then compared against height measurements using Pentagon-generated charts to determine the body fat percentage.

The bottom line for service members is that, regardless of bodyweight, you will not go to fat camp with a muscular, well-developed neck.

Last, but not least, a muscular neck screams "don't screw with me," and it will separate you from the "pec and bi warriors."

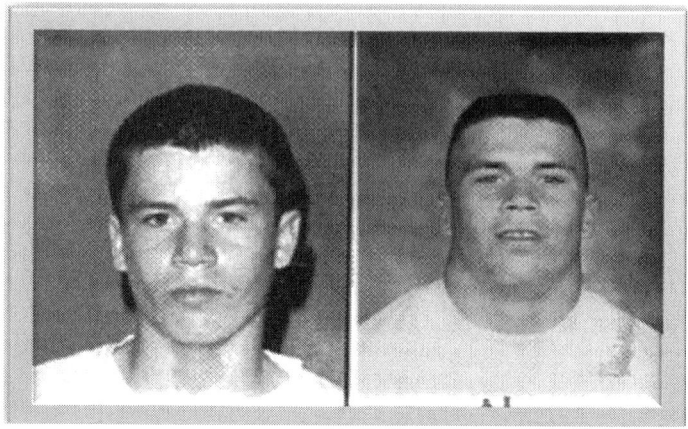

Figure 2. Co-authors, Josh Bryant and Adam benShea, started developing TST in 8th grade. Josh's neck transformation from 8th to 10th grade.

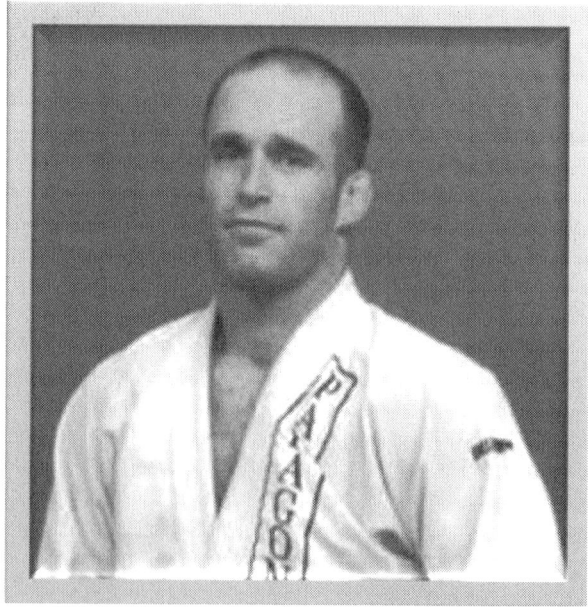

Figure 3. Adam used TST to develop neck strength for grappling

The Importance of Neck Training

How did we first hear about neck training?

Like many lessons that leave a lasting imprint, we learned about this type of training from experience. More specially, we learned from the experience of standing before powerful mentors.

Young adults are shaped by the strong people they encounter and scarred by the weak ones. Fortunately, we gravitated more to strength than weakness.

One such man of strength was an eccentric character whom we knew as Rocky. Around the beachside community where we grew up, Rocky had attained the status of a legend. He wrestled at a local high school before getting into powerlifting. Along the way, he trained in martial arts of the most esoteric variety in the Far East. Rocky spent prolonged periods of solitude and isolation in some of the more remote sections of the California mountains, where he learned to live off the land and dismiss the kind of basic bodily needs that would've crippled a lesser man. Rocky returned home with a deep and profound understanding of the universe and the energy that connects all sentient beings. Taking up residence in a trailer parked on an old homestead at the base of the foothills, Rocky was extremely selective about whom he would spend time with. The rage of his youth that led to broken bottles, bar fights, and busted-up cantinas had been tempered by age. He could, nonetheless, be cantankerous when in the company of people whose "energy" he didn't like.

For any number of reasons, he took a liking to us.

One day, shortly before our freshman year of high school, Rocky stopped by the gym on his way back from the local farmers' market (well before it was "discovered" by top bun–wearing hipsters in skinny jeans with ironic tattoos and carefully coiffed facial hair, Rocky was a voracious consumer of organic produce).

Just finished with our workout, we were walking down to the gym's parking lot as Rocky was making his way up.

Sincerely excited to see Rocky, we shouted "Hey!" with all the vigor of youth.

In sharp contrast and without a bit of irony, Rocky gave us a subtle bow and asked about our training in a quiet voice.

"Hey, fellas. It's nice to see you. How was your workout? What did you train today?"

"We did bench press and we hit some back arms," we said while pointing to our triceps to accentuate the point.

"That's good," Rocky said, nodding in understanding. "Bench press is important, essential even as a foundation for strength. And that's what you boys are building right now, a foundation. But, remember this: Don't get locked inside of the box of popular exercises. Whether you're training for combat-type sports like football, wrestling, or martial arts, or for the combative nature of living, think outside the box."

He had a magnificent life force about him, and he had our rapt attention. However, before Rocky could continue, our conversation was interrupted by the noisy din of bumping techno music coming from an SUV that was pulling into the gym parking lot.

In an instant, we witnessed a radical metamorphosis. Rocky went from a demeanor best described as "monk on the mountaintop" to having his face awash with the savage look of medieval war. Barely finished with his thoughtful assertion on training philosophy, Rocky yelled at the top of his lungs at the interlopers.

"Turn that crap music off!! It's got no soul! You've got no right to interfere with our conversation!"

As he yelled, we noticed that his neck became powerfully alive with steel rod–like tendons bouncing out from every angle.

From the SUV, the recipients of his verbal outburst emerged. There were three of them. A few years older than us and average athletes at best, they hung around town since graduation and attempted to cling to whatever status they could claim. They weren't the types to recognize the potential hazard of upsetting a guy like Rocky.

"Stuff it, old man! Nobody wants to hear your hippie music!" They responded with the impetuousness of boys who knew not that they stood before a man.

The hippie comment was an obvious reference to Rocky's long and unkempt mane of hair, his bushy beard, his bare feet (he always said that shoes interrupted his connection with the earth), and his baggy clothes.

We heard a slow whistle behind us and turned to see Sarge, an old veteran of foreign wars and long stretches in the penal system, watching with casual interest.

"Them boys are about to learn the difference between show and go," Sarge said with the calm assurance of a man who has seen enough to know the score.

Without hesitation or restraint, Rocky shed his timeworn baggy shirt like a wild thing discarding an old skin.

Following suit, the loud interlopers took off their shirts.

The bared torsos were a study in opposites. Rocky's midsection was lean and hard. His shoulders were broad, but it was his thick neck and meaty traps that served as a powerful trunk seemingly running through and supporting the center of his very being.

In contrast, the young guys had some muscle in their chests and bulges in their biceps, but their tummies were soft. Most noticeably, every one of them had pencil necks, like a stack of dimes. They had no center of strength.

Rocky walked with intent over to the trio and head-butted the guy who was clearly the aggressor—thus, applying the cardinal rule of fighting multiple opponents, which is to take the leader out first—before turning to the rest of the group, who watched their friend slump back against the SUV in dreamland.

"Now, it's your turn. Take your best shot," Rocky growled at the second guy, who had clearly lost some of the wind from his sails. "Hit me!" Rocky commanded.

Following orders, the kid reeled back, and we heard the eerie sound of knuckled bone hitting facial flesh. Rocky hardly winced at the blow.

"Again," he muttered out of the side of his mouth.

The second blow was louder than the first, but it appeared to only make Rocky angrier. It seemed that the power in Rocky's neck allowed him to endure and absorb blunt force trauma. His neck was protecting him.

"Again, like you mean it," Rocky snarled and even slapped himself to drive home the point.

The third punch had no effect on Rocky, but it left the kid shaking his hand in pain.

"I think it's broken," he muttered.

"It might be," Rocky agreed with a curt nod. "Now take your friend and get out of here before you disrupt my inner peace and really see some anger."

Nodding, the two guys picked up their friend (still dazed from the head-butt), piled into their SUV, and peeled out.

"Show muscles and go muscles, fellas. Show muscles and go muscles." We heard Sarge's deep voice behind us. "Back in the pen, we learned never to mess with a dude who had a thick neck.

Those pretty boys just learned that today."

Rocky grabbed his shirt in a smooth motion as he walked back up to us with a sense of calm returning to his countenance.

"Rocky, that was unreal," we said in genuine awe.

"Remember what we were talking about? That's the power of training outside of the box. Too many folks neglect the neck. You can't do that. It is your shield. You don't leave your shield behind. Do you know how the neck functions?"

We shook our heads.

"Do you know how to strengthen it?" Rocky asked.

Again, we shook our heads.

"Well, allow me to explain."

Neck Function

Your neck supports the weight of your head and safeguards the nerves that transmit sensory and motor information from your brain down to the rest of your body. Furthermore, your neck is extremely flexible and allows you to turn and flex in all directions.

From a training standpoint, the neck has four major functions: flexion, extension, lateral flexion, and rotation. Let's look at what each function means.

Neck flexion is a "churched up" way of saying tilting your head forward. The chief muscles involved are the longus colli, longus capitis, and sternocleidomastoid (anterior fibers).

Neck extension refers to the action of moving your chin away from your chest. The mainstay muscles in this action are the splenius capitis, semispinalis capitis, suboccipitals, trapezius, and sternocleidomastoid (posterior fibers.)

Neck lateral flexion in lay terms means tilting your head to the side. The primary muscles involved in this function are the sternocleidomastoid and scalenes.

Neck rotation simply refers to turning your head to the side. It is powered by the sternocleidomastoid, obliquus capitis (inferior & superior), rectus capitis, lateralis, longissimus capitis, splenius capitis, and the trapezius.

Most people don't even think about training their neck. The ones who do generally think about nothing beyond extension, but to truly build overall neck strength and maximize hypertrophy, it is essential to train not only extension (head back) but also flexion (head forward), rotation, and lateral flexion (side to side). This is holistic neck training for form and function.

This section on neck training should be mandatory reading for every football coach, combat sport trainer, tactical athlete, backyard brawler, and barroom bouncer. The following routine should be done thrice weekly for maximum effectiveness, but remember once is good and twice is even better.

Warm-Up

The benefits of a proper warm-up are well documented. Some of the innumerable benefits include more efficient movement patterns and increased mental readiness. Your muscles and joints also get primed. No successful lifter today forgoes this critical step. Why should you?

The following is an example of a warm-up for an intense workout.

Warm-Up
- 2 to 5 min brisk walk warm-up
- Dynamic stretch
    - Walk on toes—2 sets of 15 yards
    - Walk on heels—2 sets of 15 yards
    - Arm swings—2 sets of 10 clockwise and counterclockwise
    - Arm hugs—2 sets of 10 reps
    - Straight leg kicks—3 sets of 15 yards
    - Leg swings—2 sets of 15 reps
    - High knees—3 sets of 15 yards
    - Walking lunges—3 sets of 15 yards
    - Lateral lunges—2 sets of 10 reps (back and forth, do not hold end position)
    - Wrist sways—3 sets, 15 each way
    - Hula hip swings—2 sets of 10 clockwise and counterclockwise

To see visual examples of dynamic warm-ups, please go to the Jailhouse Strong YouTube channel. Upon completing your dynamic warm-up, start warming up for the first lifting movement of the day.

The warm-up moves in a funnel fashion from general to specific. After the general warm-up and dynamic stretching, you move to the specific phase. Warming up in a specific manner will get you mentally and physically ready to dominate the training session. So, upon completion of the warm-up described above, if you're training your neck, continue your warm-up by working your neck. We'll start with neck rotations.

Neck Rotations

To execute neck rotations, attach a band to a pole, power rack, or some other immovable object. Then place the band slightly above eye level and walk away from the immovable object so the band pulls moderately tight. From here, while maintaining good posture, rotate your head to the right so your chin is over your shoulder, then return to the center and do the exact same movement to the left side. Continue in alternating fashion for 50 reps (25 reps to each side). Do this for three sets. The first set should be the motion without band resistance. So, just rotate your head back and forth for 25 reps on each side. Set two should be with very light resistance. Finally, set three should be increasingly difficult but nowhere near a max effort. In terms of Rate of Perceived Exertion (or RPE), set two should be between 5 and 6 (on a scale of 1 to 10), and set 3 should be at a 7.

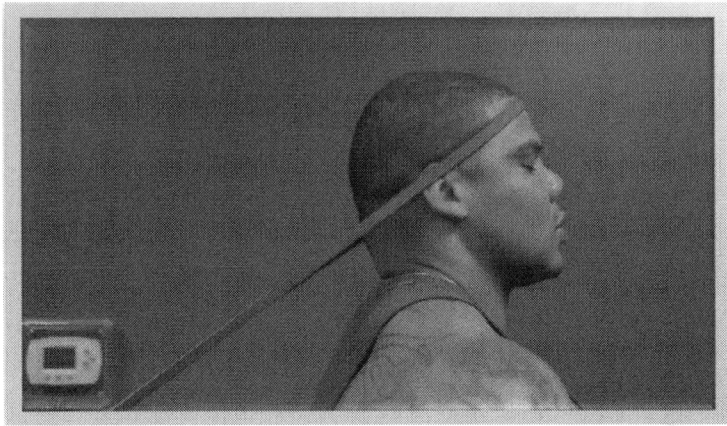

Figure 4. Neutral head starting position demonstrated by military & NFL veteran, JJ Horne.

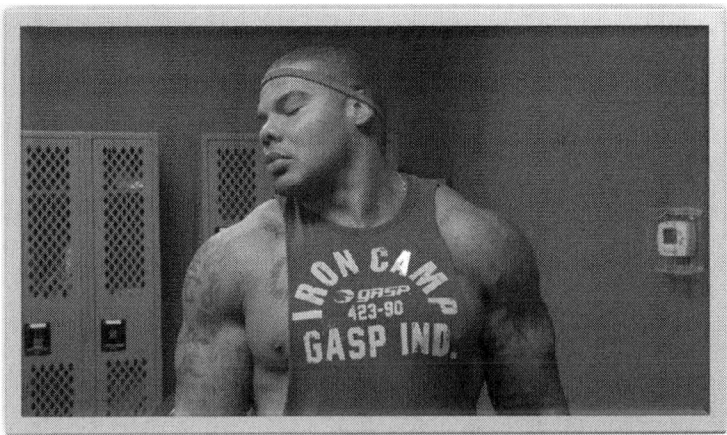

Figure 5. Turn head side to side in an alternating fashion.

Training Tips

This exercise is more of an activation warm-up exercise than a "balls-to-the-wall" heavy set; err on the side of too little resistance. To increase resistance, step farther away from the immovable object. To decrease resistance, step closer. Always start with this movement because it provides great activation and puts the finishing touches on your warm-up. This movement must be performed with strict form. Since the range of motion is short, do not cheat on it. If you don't have a band, you can do these manually resisted with your hand while following the outlined intensity guides. You can also make a band from an old bike tire (you don't have to be MacGyver to put it together).

You can continue the warm-up reps into your workout. For flexion, extension, and lateral flexion (all described below), warm up by doing one set of 15 reps of the movement you will be executing, but without weight. From there, do one set of 10 reps with 50 to 60 percent of the prescribed weight you will be using. This is the minimum, and you are welcome to do an additional one or two warm-up sets. If you don't have access to weights, any of these movements can be performed against manual resistance or a band. Enough small talk—let's get to the neck workout.

Neck Flexions

Wear a comfortable beanie, preferably a Jailhouse Strong or #GASSTATIONREADY beanie, or place a folded towel on a weight plate. Lie flat on a bench with your back flat on the bench and your feet on the floor. Place the plate on your forehead. With your head hanging off the edge of the bench, flex your head up until your chin touches your upper chest, then extend your neck backward to a comfortable stretch.

Repeat for three sets of 20 reps.

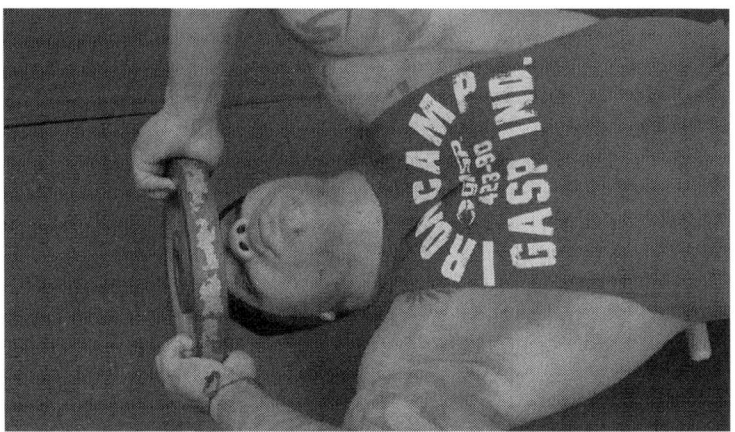

Figure 6. Bottom position of neck flexion.

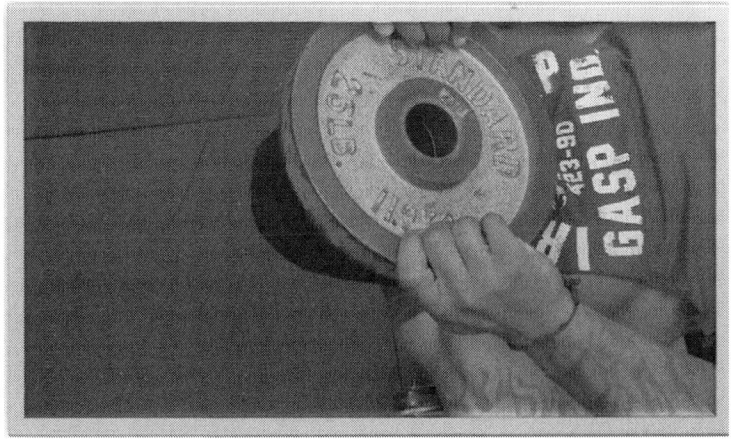

Figure 7. Contracted position of neck flexion.

Training Tips

Start off light—the weight of your head is plenty. Load the exercise by adding 2.5 pounds or less per session. Focus on strict execution of the movement, emphasizing a full range of motion. Do not be explosive, and don't jerk it on these neck movements; perform them under control.

Neck Extensions

Lie face down with your whole body straight on a flat bench while holding a weight plate behind your head. Position yourself so that your shoulders are just above the end of the bench, with your upper chest, neck, and face off the bench. This is the starting position. From here, holding the plate securely, lower your head to a comfortable stretch, then extend your head up briefly in a controlled movement and hold the extended position.

Do this for three sets of 20 reps.

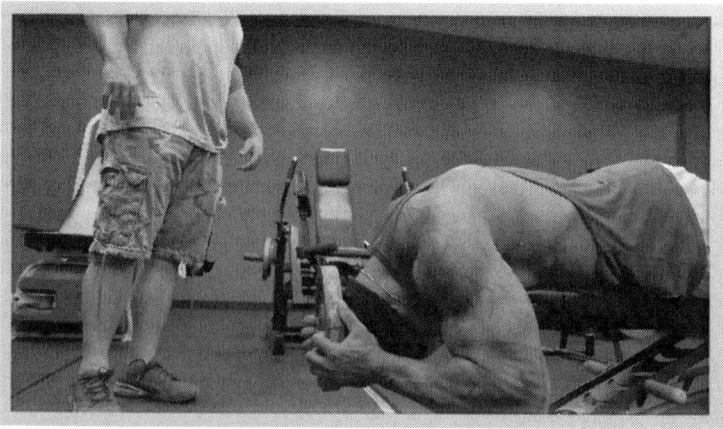

Figure 8. Bottom position of neck extension.

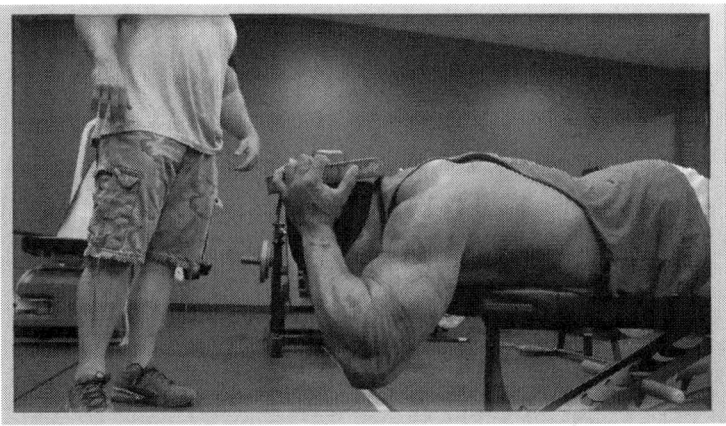

Figure 9. Contracted position of neck extension.

Training Tips
Start this exercise weightless and add a maximum of 2.5 pounds per session. Perform a full range of motion, with strict form at a controlled speed.

Neck Lateral Flexions
Place a folded towel on a weight plate. Lie on your left side on a flat bench with your legs on the floor and your left forearm on the bench. Position the weight and towel on the right side of your upper head. Hold the weight on the right side of your head with your right hand. Place your left hand on the floor for support. From here, move your head up to your right shoulder by laterally flexing your neck. Then lower your head to the left side and repeat; do the opposite for the left side.

Complete two sets of 15 for each side.

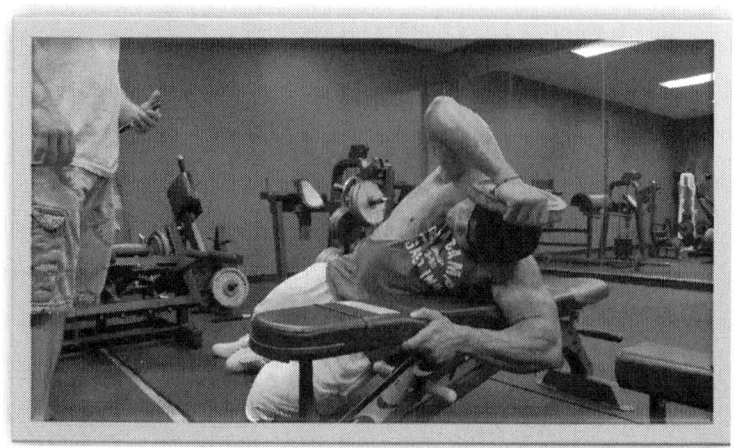

Figure 10. Bottom position of neck lateral flexion.

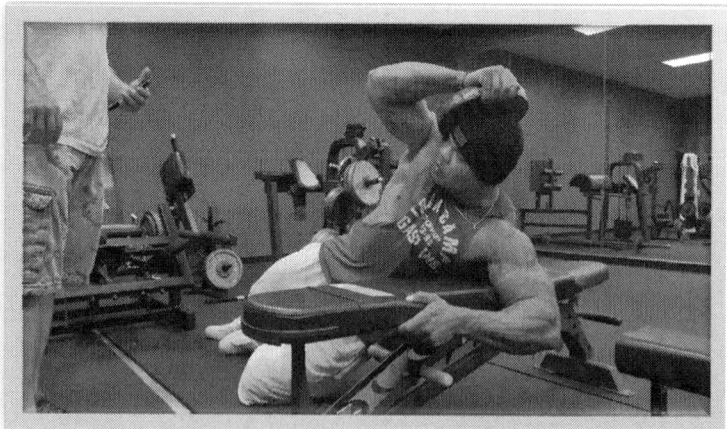

Figure 11. Contracted position of neck lateral flexion.

Training Tips

For normal-size folks, this can be done by just lying on your side on a flat bench. Keep your range of motion full and use a strict, controlled cadence. Start this exercise weightless and add a maximum of 2.5 pounds per session.

Final Thoughts

Building a strong, muscular neck can turn you from the prey to the predator. Whether the goal is staying safe in the athletic arena or preparing for an unexpected car crash, a strong neck is the answer. To get one, follow the prescribed program to a tee for a full eight weeks. Now, a truly developed neck stands on the shoulders of muscular traps. With this in mind, let's discuss how you build a broad foundation of traps to host your broad neck.

For a video demonstration of all of the following exercises, visit the Jailhouse Strong YouTube channel to view our video entitled Neck Training 101.

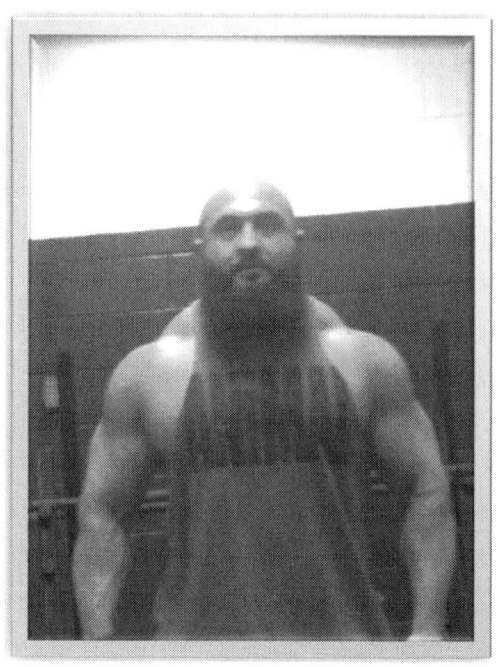

Figure 12. BJ Whitehead's trap development is in large part due to TST principles.

The Total Trap Development Program

At the local farmers' market, sculpted abs and pumped-up biceps are admired and might even get you a complimentary,

GMO-free IPA from the attractive coed working the locally sourced beer stand.

Across town, at the kick and stab bar, pumped-up biceps go unnoticed, and at worst they make you an easy target for a predator looking to make easy prey of you.

Seasoned predators know the difference between show and go muscle.

Traps are go muscles and tell any would-be assailant to look elsewhere.

Well-developed, diamond-shaped traps look like cobras coiled and ready to strike at an instant. Big traps are built by picking up heavy-ass pig iron and a lot of hard work. In contrast, visible abs can be found on starving Abercrombie models, and maybe even the local meth head.

Abs may look cool, but traps are a true strength status symbol.

When most people think about the trapezius, or "traps," they think about just the meaty part around the neck, but the reality is that the traps are a large diamond-shaped muscle bundle that goes from the base of the skull to the mid-back region. They're responsible for moving the scapula and stabilizing the entire shoulder girdle. If you don't work the whole trapezius, you'll be prone to injury. You'll also be leaving aesthetic and functional gains on the table.

The upper traps, which gym "bros" mistake as the entire muscle, elevate the scapula; the midtraps retract the scapula; and the lower traps depress the scapula. While this is an extreme crash course in anatomical trap function, you will see these various functions in our exercise section. Total trap development is our mantra!

Jailhouse Strong

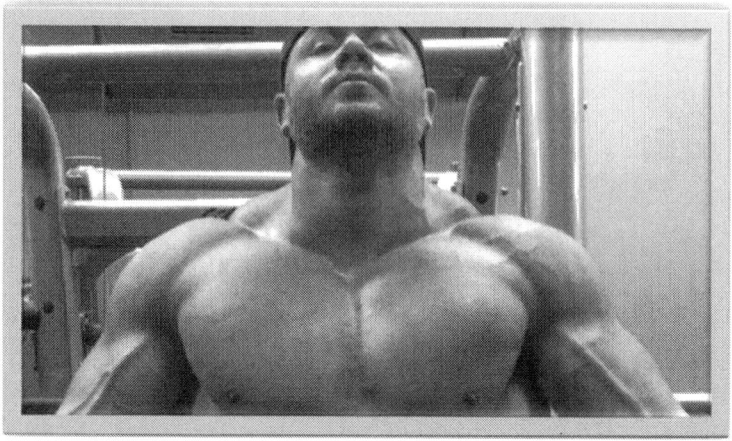

Figure 13. Tactical athlete, Tom Haviland, has built huge traps with TST Principles.

Besides the intimidation factor in sport or at the gas station at 3 a.m. (#GASSTATIONREADY), strong trap development offers a host of performance benefits, including improved posture, healthy shoulder function, greater lifting strength in any core movement or strongman event, and a greatly reduced likelihood of whiplash and/or concussions. Every football player, fighter, and combat sport athlete take note!

With this trap development program, we are starting with the supposition you are already squatting, doing deadlifts, and/or training Olympic lifts. The movements and workout described should be done in addition to your existing routine.

To make this shield-b building program as accessible as possible, we provide detailed exercises along with prescribed sets, reps, and rest interval routines for you to follow.

About the Movement: Farmer's Walk

From the big leagues to the bush leagues, the farmer's walk is a regular occurrence in strongman contests. This is why professional strongmen have the most-developed traps in the world. The farmer's walk builds muscle quickly, decreases body fat, increases strength in core lifts, improves conditioning, and is like a moving plank on steroids.

All the muscles of the upper back are hammered with the farmer's walk, but the traps take the brunt of the load! The traps are forced to work in unison to keep your shoulder blades locked together in place and to stabilize your entire shoulder girdle while under an extreme stretch. Traps thrive under both a stretch and heavy isometric tension, and the farmer's walk is king because of its ability to do both simultaneously.

The farmer's walk is becoming increasingly common inside many gyms, but it has been a longheld feature inside some of Asia's toughest martial arts regimens. For instance, many Muay Thai masters use a variation of the farmer's walk to improve their pupils' ability to endure the trauma of repetitive blows. Specifically, young trainees will hold water buckets for more than three hours. Even with this submaximal weight, the nature of the movement and the time under tension yield incredible results. Relatively skinny Thai fighters develop monster traps and improve their ability to endure strikes in the ring.

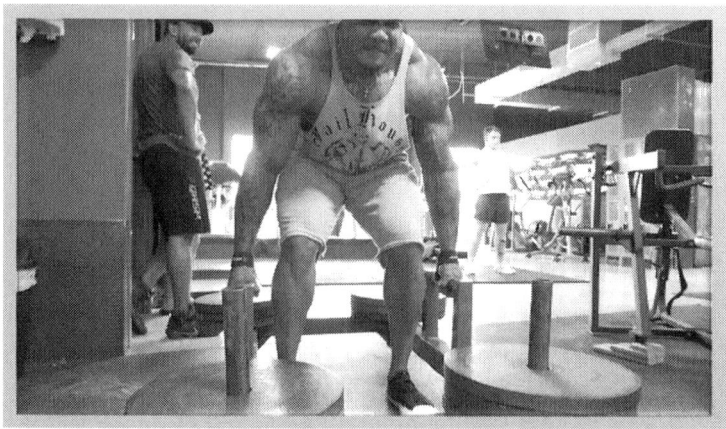

Figure 14. JJ Horne getting ready to pick up a frame carry (Farmer's Walk variation).

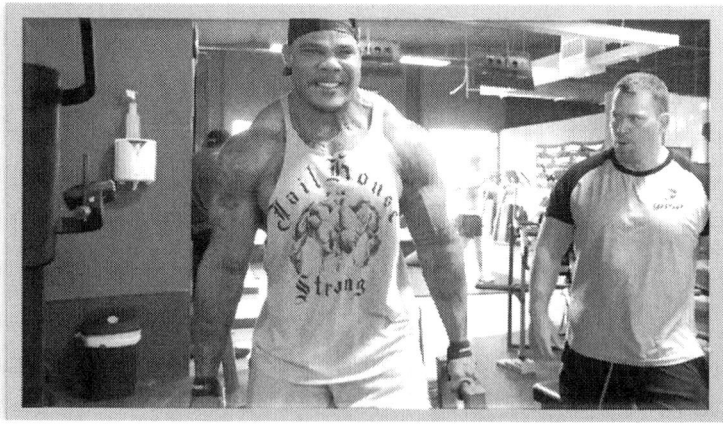

Figure 15. JJ Horne charges ahead, as coach Josh Bryant yells encouragement.

Training Tips

For the competitive strongman, the farmer's walk may be the ultimate grip test. But for trap development, we can make it even more effective! This is done by wearing straps, thus assuring that grip never limits trap development. You are going to perform farmer's walks with as much weight as possible for 30 seconds straight, covering as much distance as possible at a brisk pace. Keep in mind that total time is more important than total distance.

The farmer's walk will be performed as part of a superset with Hise shrugs; the superset will be performed three times. Start off as heavy as possible and reduce weight as needed, resting three minutes between supersets. The goal is to not exceed a 10 percent reduction in weight between supersets. So, for example, if you are performing farmer's walks with 200 pounds in one set, your goal in the subsequent set would be 180 pounds or more. A lot of weight and a lot of time under tension are going to equal a lot of trap growth.

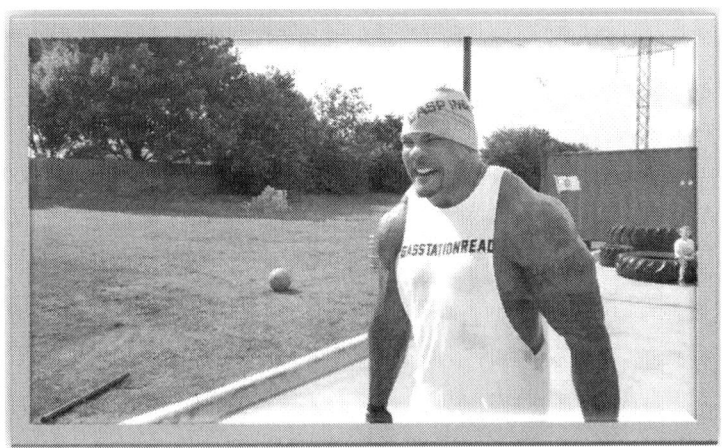

Figure 16. Farmer's Walk executed with a rickshaw implement.

Bonus Tip
If you don't have access to farmer's walk implements, some effective substitutes are a trap bar, dumbbells, a frame carry, or short barbells. Strap up and build those traps!

About the Movement: Hise Shrugs
JC Hise, the man Hise shrugs are named after, is considered by many physical culturists to be the Father of American Weightlifting. Hise, the cruel genius who spawned the 20-rep squat program, also fathered one of the most effective trap-building exercises of all time, the Hise shrug. The traditional Hise shrug is performed by putting a barbell across your shoulders like you are going to squat. However, instead of squatting, you shrug the barbell up and down.

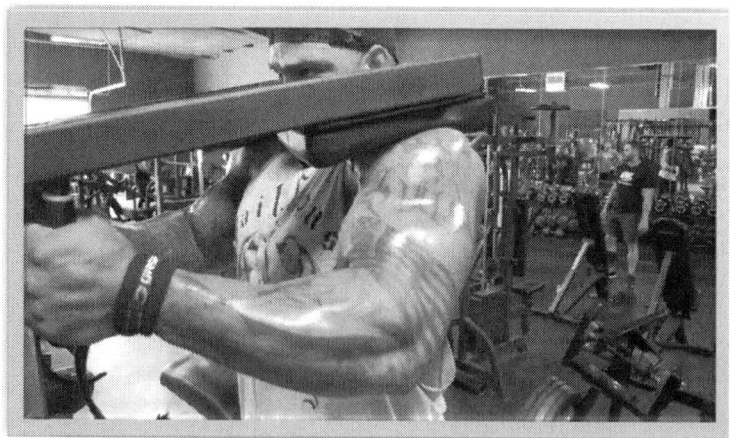

Figure 17. Hise Shrug on a standing calf raise.

Training Tips
Immediately after finishing farmer's walks, complete the superset with our modernized version of the Hise shrug on

a standing calf raise machine. This offers a huge advantage because it rests your grip and eliminates stability requirements, which were tested during farmer's walks. Therefore, you can focus on blasting your traps. Hise shrugs are performed on a standing calf raise machine by shrugging your traps up (try to touch your shoulders to your ears). Hold this top position for a three count (because of the short range of motion and to increase time under tension). Let the weight come all the way down, hold the bottom position briefly, and repeat. Go as heavy as possible, reducing weight as needed in the subsequent sets.

Bonus Tip
If you don't have a standing calf raise machine, use a hack squat machine or any other padded squat machine with neutral shoulder pads.

About the Movement: Face Pulls
In the last decade, face pulls have been one of the go-to "prehab" exercises for elite strength athletes to keep their shoulders healthy. Performed properly, this exercise can do wonders for your Neanderthal/Quasimodo posture, keep your shoulders healthy, and build the neglected midtraps.

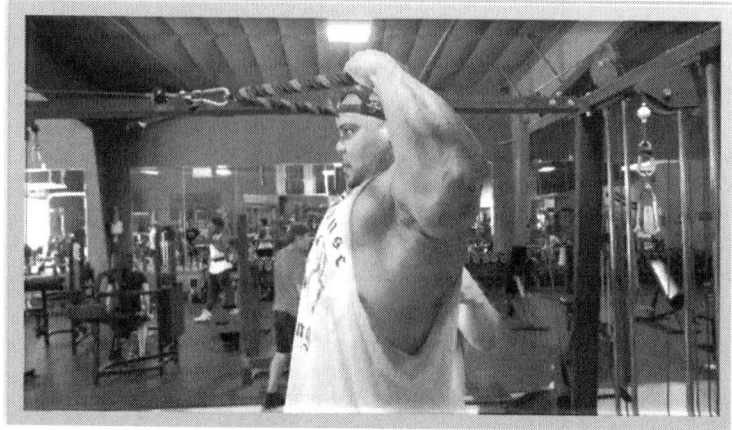

Figure 18. Face Pulls are simple but effective.

Training Tips
If you can't feel it, KILL IT! This is not a power movement; cheated, shortened range of motion might build your ego but ain't going to do diddly-squat for your mid-traps. Face pulls are performed on a pulley station with the rope at approximately neck level. Grab both ends of the rope with a neutral grip (palms facing each other). Step back so you are supporting the weight completely with your arms, which are stretched out. From here, retract the scapulae (pull your shoulder blades together) and then pull the center of the rope toward your face as you pull the ends of the rope apart and you finally finish in what looks like a double biceps pose. Hold this position for one second. Repeat for the prescribed reps.

Bonus Tip
DO NOT shrug your shoulders up. This negates the mid—trap and postural benefits.

About the Movement: Incline Dumbbell Shrugs

Most gym goers have tried dumbbell shrugs, but very few have done them on an incline; this is one of the simplest yet most effective mid-trap builders on the planet. We first learned this movement from an iron game legend, the late Paul Kelso, author of *Kelso's Shrug Book*, in a personal communication.

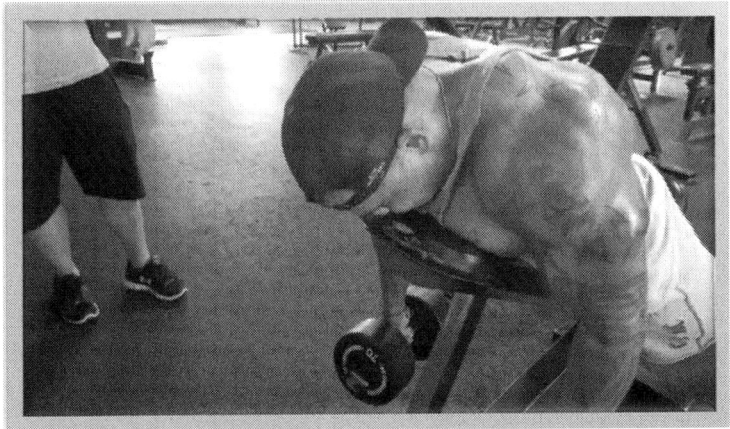

Figure 19. Incline Dumbbell Shrugs in action.

Training Tips

At most gyms, incline benches are set at approximately 4 45 degrees. For this movement, an incline shrug done that steep will primarily hit the upper traps. However, your objective is to target the neglected mid-traps. For this reason, we want to perform incline shrugs on a 30-degree incline. If you err, err to a lower angle rather than a steeper one. Lie chest down on the 30-degree incline bench and, using a neutral grip (palms facing each other), shrug up, hold the movement at the top for a three count, lower, and repeat for the prescribed reps.

Bonus Tip
If dumbbells are not available, you could perform this movement with a barbell or cables.

About the Movement: Band Y-Raises
This movement comes out of Jim Stoppani's *Encyclopedia of Muscle & Strength*. It is an exercise that has made some of the biggest, strongest men in the world scream in self-inflicted pain. The reason is because of disproportionately weak lower traps coupled with variable resistance of the band.

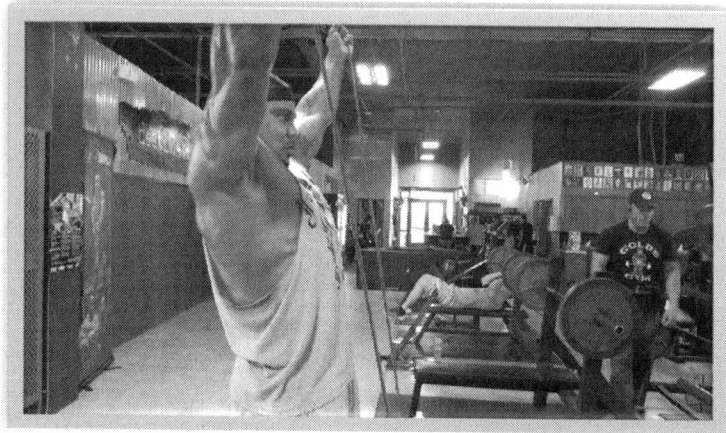

Figure 20. Band Y-Raises done with proper execution smoke the lower traps.

Training Tips
Wrap a resistance band around a stable structure so both ends of the band are right below shoulder height. Hold the ends of the band with a neutral grip (palms facing each other). Keeping your arms straight, extend your arms

straight up as high as possible so that at the end point, they form a 30-degree angle with your head. Hold this position for a two count, lower, and repeat for the prescribed reps.

Bonus Tip
Keep in mind that this is not a power movement. This is a feel movement, where you focus on pure muscle intention. So, if you don't feel this movement in your lower traps, stop and decrease the resistance (by changing bands or stepping closer to the stable structure).

As a point of reference, the opposite of a "feel movement" would be something like the deadlift, where you are looking to just move some iron.

About the Movement: Straight Arm Dip Shrugs

This is another Jim Stoppani favorite and excellent lower-trap strengthener. By strengthening your lower traps, you will ensure complete trap development, help stabilize your scapula, and decrease the likelihood of shoulder pain from strength training.

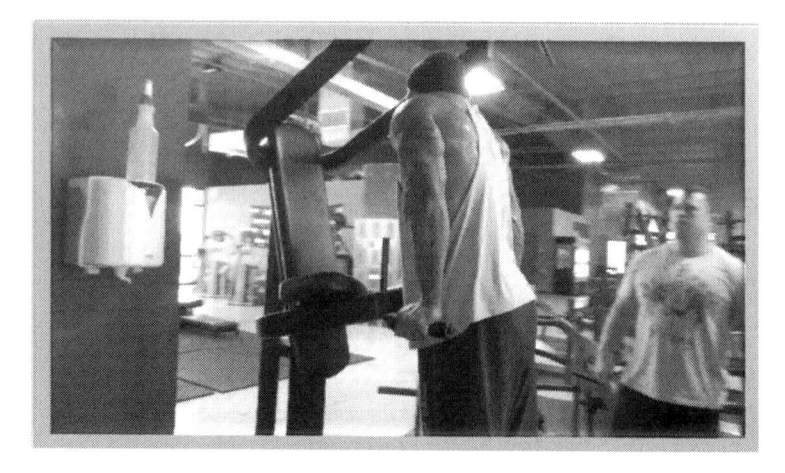

Figure 21. Keep the elbows straight on dip shrugs to maximize effectiveness.

Training Tips
Support your body on a parallel dip stand like you are going to perform traditional dips, with your arms straight and just slight of full extension. From this position, without bending your elbows, let your body sink as low as you can and then intentionally use your lower traps to pull your shoulder blades down, which will raise your body up. Attempt to raise your body as high as possible, then lower and repeat.

About the Movement: T3 Raises
This is a Charles Poliquin signature lower-trap developer.

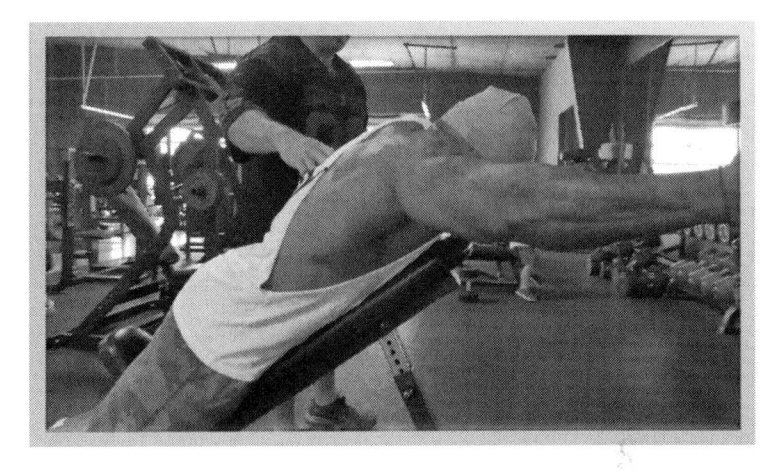

Figure 22. Thank you, Charles Poliquin, (RIP) for sharing this exercise.

Training Tips

This is not a power exercise! If you can't feel it, kill it. Lie face down on an incline bench with your arms straight and extended at your sides with a dumbbell in each hand (it is not uncommon to use five pounds or less). Initiate the movement by retracting your scapula, then raise the dumbbells out at a 45-degree angle and stop just above your head. Hold this position for three seconds. You are doing this to increase time under tension and for isometric overload.

Bonus Tip

If you are without an incline bench or dumbbells, these can be swapped out for band Y-raises.

About the Movement: One-Arm Barbell Shrugs

You read that correctly, *barbell* not dumbbell. This is an other trap-building all-star we picked up from the legendary Charles Poliquin.

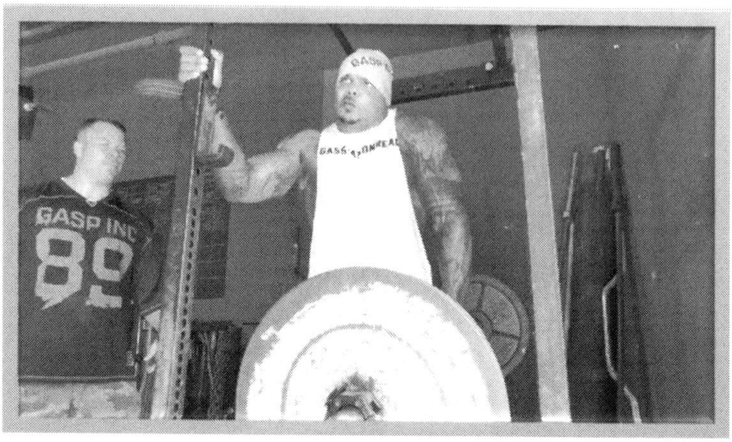

Figure 23. Brace the rack to maximize the weight you can use.

Training Tips

The one-arm barbell shrug offers a lot of advantages over traditional shrug variations. For starters, you have a much better range of motion when compared to traditional barbell shrugs. A detriment of shrugs with large dumbbells is that they create excessive amounts of friction because of cumbersome body contact. A benefit of using a barbell for shrugs, in this position, is that it keeps the shoulders neutral. An additional benefit of barbell shrugs is that they force the infraspinatus and teres minor to be recruited isometrically, as a means to prevent the barbell from moving toward the front of the body.

You will perform this movement in a power rack. Wear straps, if grip limits you. Stand to the side of the barbell and grab the middle of the barbell with your right hand while bracing your left hand on the power rack post for stability. From here, lift the barbell, shrug your right shoulder up as high as possible, and hold the top position for three seconds. Never sacrifice range of motion, but these should be performed heavy (and make sure to repeat on the other side).

Bonus Tip
This movement is a great way to increase deadlift grip strength, if done without straps.

About the Movement: Suspended Isometric Kettlebell Shrugs
This movement may look a little goofy, but the results are serious. It works because it overloads your traps concentrically, eccentrically, and isometrically. We learned it from iconic strength coach Joe DeFranco.

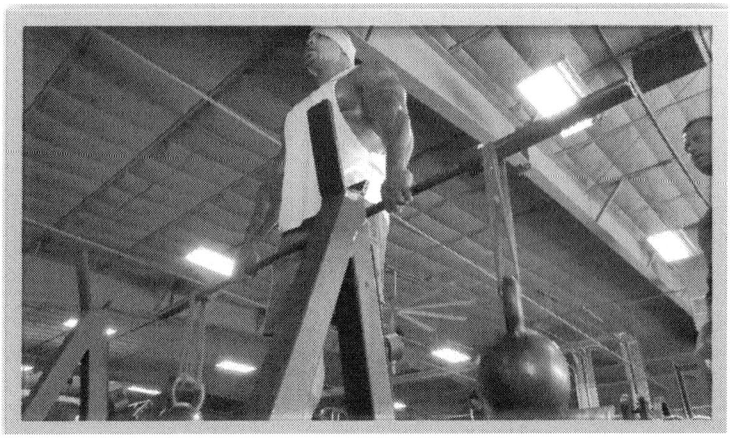

Figure 24. The start of Suspended Isometric Kettlebell Shrugs.

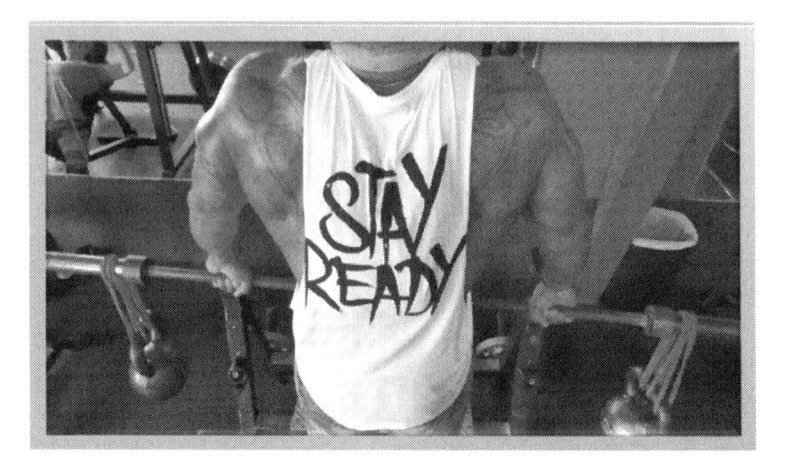

Figure 25. Rear view of Suspended Isometric Kettlebell Shrugs in action.

Training Tips

Set up a barbell in a power rack at the same height from which you would normally do a barbell shrug. Drape a doubled mini-band around the sleeves of the barbell with a kettle bell that is 10 percent of your deadlift max on each side. So, if you deadlift 400 pounds, use a 40-pound kettlebell on each side of the 45-p pound barbell. The kettlebells should be suspended off the ground, at a minimum of six inches. At this point, pick up the barbell with a wider-than-normal grip (as close to a snatch grip as you can comfortably execute); lift the barbell up and stabilize it (the suspended kettlebells will be moving). Shrug the weight up as high and explosively as possible (concentric overload), then hold the weight at the top of the movement. As you hold it, the kettlebells will bounce. It may feel like someone is pulling down on them. Fight this and hold it for three bounces (isometric overload).

Then, in a controlled fashion, lower the weight to the starting point (eccentric overload). Do this for the prescribed reps and sets. You will initially get some strange looks. Those will quickly turn to envy when they see the monstrous traps these will build!

Bonus Tip
Dumbbells will work if you don't have kettlebells, but kettlebells are best.

About the Movement: Gittleson Shrugs
This upper-trap exercise comes from legendary strength and conditioning coach Mike Gittleson. Brought in by the NFL to minimize concussions, Gittleson used this and other exercises to strengthen players' necks and traps as a first line of defense against this brain injury.

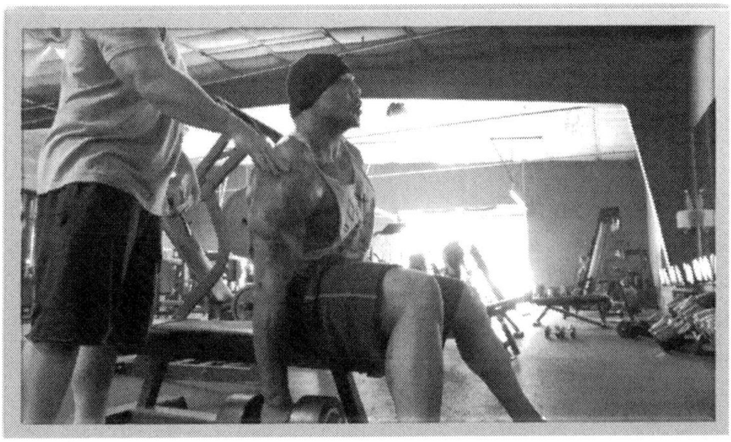

Figure 26. Stretched position of the Gittleson Shrug.

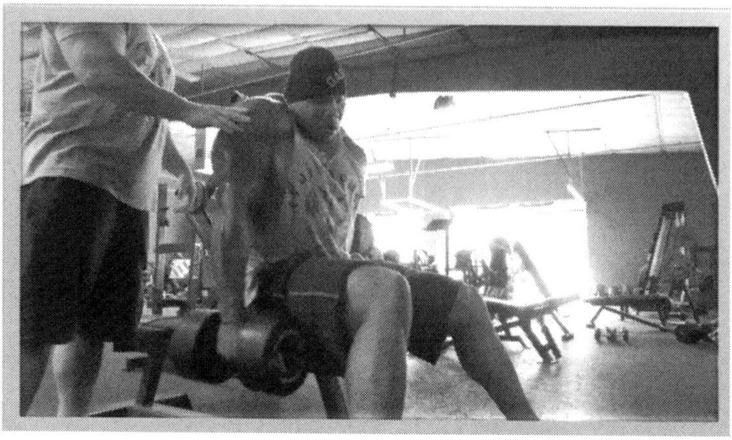

Jailhouse Strong

Figure 27. Contracted position of the Gittleson Shrug.

Training Tips
Sit on a bench and grab the side just behind your hips with the hand you're not using to do the shrugs. This will help you stay tall with good posture. Grab a dumbbell with the other hand and allow that arm to drop as low as it can toward the floor to stretch your upper trap. Shrug up as hard as possible while bringing your ear to your shoulder.

About the Movement: Half-Mile Carry
This will not only build your traps but also develop your testicular fortitude. You are going to take a pair of dumbbells and walk a half mile as fast as you can. For weight, start with 10 percent of your deadlift max.

Training Tips
Keep track of your time as you do this finisher. Do not let your grip limit you. Slap on the strap on. Ahem, as in go heavy and use straps. Drop weight, if it is necessary to finish the half mile.

The Jailhouse Strong Tactical Shield Training (TST) Program

Rome wasn't built in a day, but you can bet your ass they were laying bricks daily. Emaciated male (we use the term loosely) Abercrombie models have abs, but a well-developed neck and traps seep masculine virility and have an omnipresent aura of hard work, functional strength, toughness, and if we meet mano y mano on the lower field or the kick stab bar, I am kicking the shit out of you.

In the Jailhouse Strong Tactical Shield Training (TST) program, we have laid out exactly what to do to build your traps and neck.

The TST program can be a four day program, with up to three days for neck work and one day for traps. Beyond that, we include clear instructions for a complete strength regimen.

For those of you that are always hungry for more training, we also offer extra "meat" or movements to strengthen your neck.

Make the TST program work for you. Do it your way.

You can follow your own strength program and implement two to three days of our neck program and one day of the traps program. Or you can follow what is laid out below in our eightweek TST program, every exercise, set, rep, weight, and rest interval.

The exercise selection, intensity, and volume prescribed are a synergistic prescription that optimizes functional strength, jaw-dropping hypertrophy, and the optimal hormonal response. With the TST program, you have the means to develop your traps and neck, which might put you out of the running for the next Gillette ad, but you'll also be less likely to get sucker punched next time you're in a seedy Hong Kong dive bar.

Here is Day 1; explicit instructions on exercise execution are listed previously in the manual.

Day 1/Week 1

Exercise	Sets	Reps	Weight	Rest Interval
Farmer's Walk (superset with Hise shrugs)	3	30 sec straight	Heavy as possible	180 sec
Hise Shrugs	3	10	Heavy as possible	
Face Pulls	3	12	Heavy as possible	60 sec
Incline Dumbbell Shrugs	3	12	Heavy as possible	60 sec
T3 Raises	3	8	Heavy as possible	60 sec
Band Y-Raises	3	12	Maximum resistance	40 sec

Additional Notes
- Aside from the farmer's walk, the objective in all exercises is to increase weight weekly but never at the

expense of technique. Aim for an increase of 5 to 10 percent weekly.

Day 1/Week 2

Exercise	Sets	Reps	Weight	Rest Interval
Farmer's Walk (superset with Hise shrugs)	3	34 seconds straight	Heavy as possible	180 sec
Hise Shrugs	3	12	Heavy as possible	
Face Pulls	3	12	Heavy as possible	60 sec
Incline Dumbbell Shrugs	3	12	Heavy as possible	60 sec
T3 Raises	3	8	Heavy as possible	60 sec
Band Y-Raises	3	12	Maximum resistance	40 sec

Day 1/Week 3

Exercise	Sets	Reps	Weight	Rest Interval
Farmer's Walk (superset with Hise shrugs)	3	34 seconds straight	Heavy as possible	180 sec

Exercise	Sets	Reps	Weight	Rest Interval
Hise Shrugs	3	12	Heavy as possible	
Face Pulls	3	12	Heavy as possible	60 sec
Incline Dumbbell Shrugs	3	12	Heavy as possible	60 sec
T3 Raises	3	8	Heavy as possible	60 sec
Band Y-Raises	3	12	Maximum resistance	40 sec

Day 1/Week 4

Exercise	Sets	Reps	Weight	Rest Interval
Farmer's Walk (superset with Hise shrugs)	3	42 seconds straight	Heavy as possible	180 sec
Hise Shrugs	3	15	Heavy as possible	
Face Pulls	3	12	Heavy as possible	60 sec
Incline Dumbbell Shrugs	3	15	Heavy as possible	60 sec

Exercise	Sets	Reps	Weight	Rest Interval
T3 Raises	3	8	Heavy as possible	60 sec
Band Y-Raises	3	12	Maximum resistance	40 sec

Day 1/Week 5

Exercise	Sets	Reps	Weight	Rest Interval
Farmer's Walk	3	44 seconds straight	Heavy as possible	180 sec
Face Pulls (superset with straight arm dip shrugs)	3	12	Heavy as possible	60 sec
Straight Arm Dip Shrugs	3	15	Heavy as possible	70 sec
Suspended Isometric Kettlebell Shrugs	3	6	Heavy as possible	90 sec
Half-Mile Carry	1	Half mile	Heavy as possible	

Additional Notes
- With farmer's walks, each week you should use the same weight as the week before and focus on keeping up with the time increases. After the fifth week, the

time decreases and you should focus on increasing the weight for the next level of development. You can increase weight 5 to 10 percent weekly.
- Start half-mile carries with 10 percent of your one-rep deadlift max. So, for example, if you deadlift 400 pounds, start with 40 pounds total (i.e., 20 pounds in each hand) and increase five to ten pounds weekly.

Day 1/Week 6

Exercise	Sets	Reps	Weight	Rest Interval
Farmer's Walk	3	36 seconds straight	Heavy as possible	180 sec
Face Pulls (superset with straight arm dip shrugs)	3	15	Heavy as possible	60 sec
Straight Arm Dip Shrugs	3	18	Heavy as possible	70 sec
Suspended Isometric Kettlebell Shrugs	3	6	Heavy as possible	90 sec
Half-Mile Carry	1	Half mile	Heavy as possible	

Day 1/Week 7

Exercise	Sets	Reps	Weight	Rest Interval
Farmer's Walk	3	30 seconds straight	Heavy as possible	180 sec
Face Pulls (superset with straight arm dip shrugs)	3	15	Heavy as possible	60 sec
Straight Arm Dip Shrugs	3	20	Heavy as possible	70 sec
Suspended Isometric Kettlebell Shrugs	3	6	Heavy as possible	90 sec
Half-Mile Carry	1	Half mile	Heavy as possible	

Day 1/Week 8

Exercise	Sets	Reps	Weight	Rest Interval
Farmer's Walk	3	30 seconds straight	Heavy as possible	180 sec

Exercise	Sets	Reps	Weight	Rest Interval
Face Pulls (superset with straight arm dip shrugs)	3	15	Heavy as possible	60 sec
Straight Arm Dip Shrugs	3	20	Heavy as possible	60 sec
Suspended Isometric Kettlebell Shrugs	3	6	Heavy as possible	90 sec
Half-Mile Carry	1	Half mile	Heavy as possible	

Additional Notes
- With straight arm dip shrugs and suspended isometric kettlebell shrugs, it is important to keep good technique. However, since they are unfamiliar exercises and your muscles aren't usually worked in this way, you may progress more quickly. It is not uncommon to progress 10 percent or more each week.

Day 2 Neck Workout

Exercise	Sets	Reps	Weight	Rest Interval
Neck Rotations	2	25 each way	See notes	45 sec
Neck Flexions	3	20	See notes	60 sec

Exercise	Sets	Reps	Weight	Rest Interval
Neck Extensions	3	20	See notes	60 sec
Neck Lateral Flexions	2	15 each way	See notes	30 sec between sides

In the spirit of the late, great Joe Weider's muscle priority training, always start Day 2 with the above neck routine. For explicit instructions on how to execute each movement and how to progress with each weight, reread the neck exercise section of the manuscript.

Day 2/Week 1

Exercise	Sets	Reps	Weight	Rest Interval
Bench Presses	2	Rest pause	72.5%, 65%	120 sec
Seal Dumbbell Rows	8	8	20 rep max	30 sec
Overhead Presses	6	1	75%	30 sec
Neutral-Grip Pull-Ups	8	3	10 reps max	30 sec
Overhead Barbell Shrugs	8	8	Heavy as possible	30 sec
Dumbbell Pause Floor Triceps Extensions	8	8	20 rep max	30 sec

Additional Notes
- For all movements (aside from the ones with specific weights listed), attempt to progress five pounds or more weekly while keeping great technique. Never increase weight at the expense of form.
- Rest Pause is a term that means completing reps until one shy of failure. Then rest 20 seconds. Complete reps again until one shy of failure. Rest for 30 seconds, and for a third time complete reps until one shy of failure. So, one rest pause set is really three mini sets.

Day 2/Week 2

Exercise	Sets	Reps	Weight	Rest Interval
Bench Presses	2	Rest pause	75%, 65%	120 sec
Seal Dumbbell Rows	8	8	20 rep max	30 sec
Overhead Presses	6	1	77.5%	30 sec
Neutral-Grip Pull-Ups	9	3	10 reps max	30 sec
Overhead Barbell Shrugs	8	8	Heavy as possible	30 sec
Dumbbell Pause Floor Triceps Extensions	8	8	20 rep max	30 sec

Day 2/Week 3

Exercise	Sets	Reps	Weight	Rest Interval
Bench Presses	2	Rest pause	75%, 70%	120 sec
Seal Dumbbell Rows	8	8	20 rep max	30 sec
Overhead Presses	6	1	80%	30 sec
Neutral-Grip Pull-Ups	10	3	10 reps max	30 sec
Overhead Barbell Shrugs	8	8	Heavy as possible	30 sec
Dumbbell Pause Floor Triceps Extensions	8	8	20 rep max	30 sec

Day 2/Week 4

Exercise	Sets	Reps	Weight	Rest Interval
Bench Presses	2	5	70%	120 sec
Seal Dumbbell Rows	8	4	20 rep max	30 sec
Overhead Presses	5	1	80%	30 sec

Exercise	Sets	Reps	Weight	Rest Interval
Neutral-Grip Pull-Ups	3	3	10 reps max	30 sec
Overhead Barbell Shrugs	8	4	Same weight as Week 1	30 sec
Dumbbell Pause Floor Triceps Extensions	8	4	20 rep max	30 sec

Day 2/Week 5

Exercise	Sets	Reps	Weight	Rest Interval
Bench Presses	2	Rest Pause	77.5%, 70%	120 sec
Seal Dumbbell Rows	4	8	Heavy as possible	60 sec
Overhead Presses	5	1	82.5%	30 sec
Straight Arm Pulldowns	4	12	Heavy as possible	60 sec
Seated Dumbbell Shrugs	8	8	Heavy as possible	30 sec
Tate Presses	4	12	Heavy as possible	60 sec

Day 2/Week 6

Exercise	Sets	Reps	Weight	Rest Interval
Bench Presses	2	Rest Pause	80%, 70%	120 sec
Seal Dumbbell Rows	4	7	Heavy as possible	60 sec
Overhead Presses	4	1	85%	45 sec
Straight Arm Pulldowns	4	14	Heavy as possible	30 sec
Seated Dumbbell Shrugs	8	8	Heavy as possible	30 sec
Tate Presses	4	15	Heavy as possible	60 sec

Day 2/Week 7

Exercise	Sets	Reps	Weight	Rest Interval
Bench Presses	2	Rest Pause	80%, 75%	120 sec
Seal Dumbbell Rows	4	6	Heavy as possible	60 sec

Exercise	Sets	Reps	Weight	Rest Interval
Overhead Presses	3	1	87.5%	45 sec
Straight Arm Pulldowns	4	15	Heavy as possible	30 sec
Seated Dumbbell Shrugs	8	8	Heavy as possible	30 sec
Tate Presses	4	10	Heavy as possible	60 sec

Day 2/Week 8

Exercise	Sets	Reps	Weight	Rest Interval
Bench Presses	2	5	70%	120 sec
Seal Dumbbell Rows	3	6	75% of Week 7 weight	60 sec
Overhead Presses	3	1	75%	45 sec
Straight Arm Pulldowns	3	12	75% of Week 7 weight	30 sec
Seated Dumbbell Shrugs	3	8	Week 5 weight	30 sec
Tate Presses	3	10	75% of Week 7 weight	60 sec

Day 3 Neck Workout

Exercise	Sets	Reps	Weight	Rest Interval
Neck Rotations	2	25 each way	See notes	45 sec
Neck Flexions	3	20	See notes	60 sec
Neck Extensions	3	20	See notes	60 sec
Neck Lateral Flexions	2	15 each way	See notes	30 sec between sides

- In the spirit of the late, great Joe Weider's muscle priority training, always start Day 3 with the above neck routine. For explicit instructions on how to execute each movement and how to progress with each weight, reread the neck exercise section of the manuscript.

Day 3/Week 1

Exercise	Sets	Reps	Weight	Rest Interval
Squats	6	5	70%	120 sec
Deadlifts	12	1	75%	30 sec
Leg Curls	10	2	12-rep max	20 sec
Leg Presses	2	20	Heavy as possible	90 sec
Gittleson Shrugs	3	6	Heavy as possible	45 sec

Additional Notes
- Any squat variation from the following list is okay: front squats, high bar squats, safety squats, Hatfield overload squats, or belt squats
- Acceptable deadlift variations are trap bar deadlifts, block pulls, or snatch grip deadlifts
- For all movements (aside from ones with specific weights listed), attempt to progress five pounds or more weekly while keeping great technique. Never increase weight at the expense of form.

Day 3/Week 2

Exercise	Sets	Reps	Weight	Rest Interval
Squats	7	5	70%	120 sec
Deadlifts	13	1	75%	30 sec
Leg Curls	10	3	12-rep max	20 sec
Leg Presses	2	18	Heavy as possible	90 sec
Gittleson Shrugs	3	6	Heavy as possible	45 sec

Day 3/Week 3

Exercise	Sets	Reps	Weight	Rest Interval
Squats	8	5	70%	120 sec
Deadlifts	15	1	75%	30 sec
Leg Curls	10	3	12-rep max	15 sec

Exercise	Sets	Reps	Weight	Rest Interval
Leg Presses	2	16	Heavy as possible	90 sec
Gittleson Shrugs	3	7	Heavy as possible	45 sec

Day 3/Week 4

Exercise	Sets	Reps	Weight	Rest Interval
Squats	6	2	70%	120 sec
Deadlifts	5	1	75%	30 sec
Leg Curls	3	3	10-rep max	30 sec
Gittleson Shrugs	3	7	Heavy as possible	45 sec

Day 3/Week 5

Exercise	Sets	Reps	Weight	Rest Interval
Squats	9	5	70%	120 sec
Deadlifts	10	1	80%	35 sec
One-Leg Dumbbell RDLs	2	5	12-rep max	45 sec
Sled Drag Backwards	2	100 feet	Heavy as possible	90 sec
Gittleson Shrugs	3	8	Heavy as possible	45 sec

Day 3/Week 6

Exercise	Sets	Reps	Weight	Rest Interval
Squats	10	5	70%	120 sec
Deadlifts	8	1	82.5%	40 sec
One-Leg Dumbbell RDLs	2	5	12-rep max	45 sec
Sled Drag Backwards	2	100 feet	Heavy as possible	90 sec
Gittleson Shrugs	3	8	Heavy as possible	45 sec

Day 3/Week 7

Exercise	Sets	Reps	Weight	Rest Interval
Squats	5	5	80%	150 sec
Deadlifts	6	1	85%	45 sec
One-Leg Dumbbell RDLs	2	5	12-rep max	45 sec
Sled Drag Backwards	2	100 feet	Heavy as possible	90 sec
Gittleson Shrugs	3	9	Heavy as possible	45 sec

Day 3/Week 8

Exercise	Sets	Reps	Weight	Rest Interval
Squats	2	5	70%	120 sec
Deadlifts	5	1	75%	30 sec
One-Leg Dumbbell RDLs	2	3	70% of Week 7	30 sec
Gittleson Shrugs	3	10	Heavy as possible	45 sec

Day 4/Neck Workout

Exercise	Sets	Reps	Weight	Rest Interval
Neck Rotations	2	25 each way	See notes	45 sec
Neck Flexions	3	20	See notes	60 sec
Neck Extensions	3	20	See notes	60 sec
Neck Lateral Flexions	2	15 each way	See notes	30 sec between sides

In the spirit of the late, great Joe Weider's muscle priority training, always start Day 4 with the above neck routine. For explicit instructions on how to execute each movement and how to progress with each weight, reread the neck exercise section of the manuscript. This day is completely optional. It can be used to focus on any other existing weak points, be they technique or other muscle groups that need additional attention. For the true Shield Warrior, Day 4 can also be Day 1 done all over again. The difference is that you will reduce all prescribed weights by 30 percent. For example, a farmer's walk with 200 pounds would be executed with 140 pounds.

Day 4

Exercise	Sets	Reps	Weight	Rest Interval
Neutral-Grip Pull-Ups	3	10	15-rep max	60 sec
Pec Deck Rear Delt Flys	3	15	20-rep max	60 sec
Walking Lunges	3	20 yards	Moderate	60 sec
Kettlebell Swings	3	12	Moderate	60 sec
Reverse Curls	3	15	20-rep max	60 sec
Triceps Pushdowns	3	15	20-rep max	60 sec

Extra Meat for Extra Training

Still hungry for more training? Here are isometric and combat functional training options for additional neck strengthening.

These are options which can be utilized in addition to the program described above and/or on off days.

Zen and the Lost Art of Isometrics
Isometric training is a great way to develop increased neck strength without placing an undue amount of stress on your body.

Isometrics for the Front Neck Muscles
Staying in a neutral position, put one or both hands on top of your forehead. Then, with maximum effort, push your forehead against your palm(s). To match the resistance of your head, your palms should allow for no movement of the head, thus creating a static hold (isometric contraction). Hold this for 7 to 10 seconds and repeat 5 to 10 times. This can also be done against an immovable object or resistance provided by a partner.

Isometrics for the Back Neck Muscles
Start with the same position as above, but now place both hands behind the top of your head to provide resistance for the isometric contraction. Now press the back of your head, with maximum effort, against the resistance of your hands, which again should allow for no movement to take place. Hold this for 7 to 10 seconds and repeat 5 to 10 times. As before, this can also be done against an immovable object or resistance provided by a partner.

Isometrics for the Side Neck Muscles (Neck Lateral Flexors)
Commence this old-time strongman favorite with your palm against the right side of your head.

Push your head, with maximum effort, against your palm(s) so that no movement takes place.

Hold this for 7 to 10 seconds and repeat 4 to 6 times (complete on the opposite side as well).

This can also be done against an immovable object or resistance provided by a partner.

Neck Training for Combat Sports

For centuries, combat athletes from ancient Pankration competitors to modern MMA fighters have used neck exercises to protect themselves and improve their ability to apply martial techniques. These movements require minimal equipment (a resistance band or bike tube), and they can be done just about anywhere from a playground on South Beach to a border town motel room in El Paso.

Now, there are plenty of examples of neck training inside of the realm of combat sports that are popular but potentially damaging. The nature of training in martial arts, grappling, boxing, and combat sports is that it can take a toll on your body over time.

However, with the correct training regimen, you maximize the benefits of combat training and minimize the detriments. Rather than compression exercises that place undue and unnecessary stress on your body, in general, and your neck, in particular, we include the following classic combat training exercises to give you a comprehensive training program that places minimal stress on the body.

In fact, these movements can be done as part of a warm-up or as active recovery on off days.

Nod If You Want a Stronger Neck

A staple training technique of Brazilian jiu-jitsu and judo fighters that evolved out of some of Brazil's toughest *favelas* (ghettos), this is a low-impact movement that offers noticeable results in function and form (i.e., sharpening your facial features).

Lie on your back. Lift your head and bring your chin to your chest for a set of 40 repetitions. Keep your head off the mat and look to your left for a set of 40. Repeat to the right. Keeping your head raised off the mat, touch your left ear to your left shoulder for 40 repetitions. Repeat to your right. Go through this circuit 2 to 3 times; you will be amazed at the difficulty and effectiveness.

This movement is effective for strengthening the muscles around the neck, which aids grapplers in the clinch and protects against choke attempts. It also tones the jaw, helping construct a classically handsome square jaw line and getting rid of an ugly double chin.

Walk Tall

We first learned about this movement after seeing it performed by Brazilian jiu-jitsu legend Rickson Gracie in the 1999 documentary *Choke*. Attach one side of a resistance band (a deflated bike tube or an elastic band will work) to an immovable object (e.g., the bar of a cell or a bunk bed) and loop the other side around your forehead. With good posture, walk forward until the band becomes taut. Then, incrementally, continue to move forward. This unorthodox training technique will increase your neck, and overall, strength. This can be done in very limited space. We recommend 2 to 3 sets of 30 to 50 seconds of continuous moving forward tension, followed by a rest interval of the same time to twice as long. Concentrate on maintaining good posture, not on covering a certain distance with poor posture. For variety, this movement can be performed walking backward and by sliding/shuffling laterally (sideways).

Conclusion

While it was the Spartans who stressed the importance of clinging to your shield, you don't have to be putting down a Helot revolt or marching against a rival Greek city state to start polishing your shield.

The contemporary tactical athlete needs a powerful neck as much as the ancient Spartan needed his shield.

A stronger neck will improve your performance in combat sports, decrease potential injury during an obstacle race, and reduce some of the physical stress associated with military deployment.

A tactical athlete is only as strong as arsenal. With the TST program, you now have the means to fortify your shield.

Whether you are off to a combat zone in the dry central Eurasian steppe, a local grappling tournament, or a brief trip to the perpetually volatile fish market in Cairo, don't leave home without your shield.

Printed by Amazon Italia Logistica S.r.l.
Torrazza Piemonte (TO), Italy